# AIP (Autoimmune Paleo) Diet

*A Beginner's Step-by-Step Guide and Review*

*With Recipes and a Meal Plan*

Copyright © 2019 Brandon Gilta

All rights reserved. No portion of this book may be reproduced in any form without permission from the publisher, except as permitted by U.S. copyright law.

Disclaimer

By reading this disclaimer, you are accepting the terms of the disclaimer in full. If you disagree with this disclaimer, please do not read the book. The content in this book is provided for informational and educational purposes only.

This book is not intended to be a substitute for the original work of this diet plan. At most, this book is intended to be beginner's supplement to the original work for this diet plan and never act as a direct substitute. This book, is an overview, review, and commentary of the facts of that diet plan.

All product names, diet plans, or names used in this book are for identification purposes only and are property of their respective owners. Use of these names does not imply endorsement. All other trademarks cited herein are property of their respective owners.

None of the information in this book should be accepted as independent medical or other professional advice.

The information in the books has been compiled from various sources that are deemed reliable. It has been analyzed and summarized to the best of the Author's ability, knowledge, and belief. However, the Author cannot guarantee the accuracy and thus should not be held liable for any errors.

You acknowledge and agree that the Author of this book will not be held liable for any damages, costs, expenses, resulting from the application of the information in this book, whether directly or indirectly. You acknowledge and agree that you assume all risk and responsibility for any action you undertake in response to the information in this book.

You acknowledge and agree that by continuing to read this book, you will (where applicable, appropriate, or necessary) consult a qualified medical professional on this information. The information in this book is not intended to be any sort of medical advice and should not be used in lieu of any medical advice by a licensed and qualified medical professional.

Always seek the advice of your physician or another qualified health provider with any issues or questions you might have regarding any sort of medical condition. Do not ever disregard any qualified professional medical advice or delay seeking that advice because of anything you have read in this book.

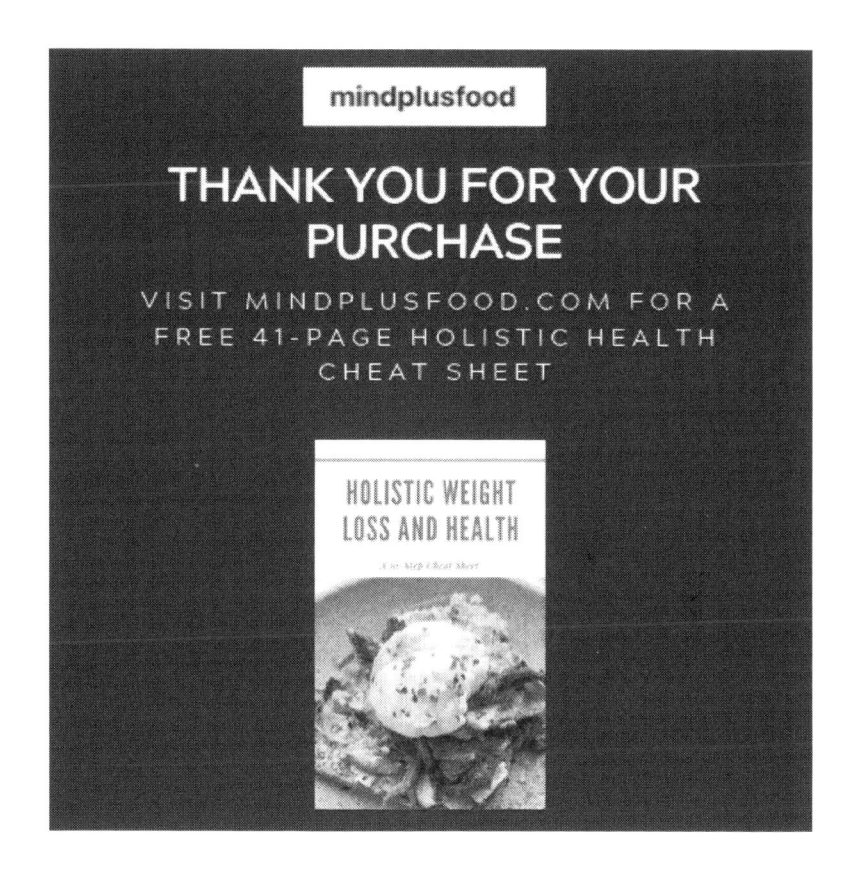

**mindplusfood**

# THANK YOU FOR YOUR PURCHASE

VISIT MINDPLUSFOOD.COM FOR A FREE 41-PAGE HOLISTIC HEALTH CHEAT SHEET

**HOLISTIC WEIGHT LOSS AND HEALTH**

# Table of Contents

*Introduction* ............................................................. 5
*Chapter 1 – About the Diet* ...................................... 7
*Chapter 2 – Gut Matters* ........................................ 13
*Chapter 3 – Week 1* ................................................ 16
*Chapter 4 – Week 2* ................................................ 19
*Chapter 5 - Week 3* ................................................ 22
*Chapter 6 – Week 4 and beyond* ........................... 27
*Chapter 7- Selected Recipes* .................................. 29
    Instant Pot Bone Broth ..................................... 29
    Roasted Pork Chops .......................................... 31
    Roasted Chicken Thighs ................................... 34
    Turmeric Tea ..................................................... 35
    Blackberry Cobbler ........................................... 37
    Cauliflower Rice ................................................ 39
    Asian Stir-Fry .................................................... 40
    Ramen Noodle Soup ......................................... 42
    Green Curry Paste ............................................ 45
    Thai Green Curry .............................................. 46
    Salmon Soup ..................................................... 49
*Chapter 8- My Review and Analysis of the Diet* ............................................................................. 53
*Conclusion* .............................................................. 56

# Introduction

I want to thank you and congratulate you for getting this guide.

If you are struggling with autoimmune diseases such as rheumatoid arthritis you might be curious about alternative ways of managing your symptoms.

While medications may dull chronic pain, they sometimes come with unpleasant side effects. Also known as the autoimmune protocol diet, the autoimmune paleo (AIP) diet offers one way of helping reduce your symptoms by addressing one of their potential causes.

The AIP diet provides people with autoimmune diseases an opportunity to manage chronic pain by eliminating specific type of foods that are thought to cause or worsen inflammation throughout the body. In addition, the diet also incorporates many different types of food that could help reduce joint inflammation and soothe pain, including those rich in healthy omega-3 fatty acids. Some patients have reported a reduce the need for their pain medications and significant improvements in their quality of life.

This book provides a comprehensive and concise look at the benefits of the AIP diet and offers a step-by-step guide for meal planning. It also judges the merits of the diet based on the available evidence and shares a few important steps to remember when trying this diet.

Thanks again for getting this book. I hope you enjoy it!

# Chapter 1 – About the Diet

Identified as a variant of the much more familiar paleo diet, the AIP diet employs a much more refined and restrictive approach to meal planning. The AIP diet is focused on preventing and addressing leaky gut syndrome. Certain types of food are thought to contribute to the disorder, which can lead to or worsen the progression of autoimmune diseases, among them rheumatoid arthritis.

Both paleo diet and the AIP diet were based on the work of Dr. Loren Cordain, PhD, who believed that a diet low in carbohydrates and rich in vegetables, proteins, and healthy sources of fat are closer to humans' natural diets and thus significantly healthier for the human body.

Further developments on the AIP diet were made by author Robb Wolfe, who outlined it as an elimination diet, and Dr. Sarah Ballantyne, PhD, who did extensive research on the science behind it. Dr. Ballantyne discussed the diet and its benefits extensively in her book *The Paleo Approach*.

Because it did not involve cutting out many popular meat dishes, the paleo diet became a popular way of managing weight. This isn't just your average weight loss diet; it is meant to be part of a comprehensive pain management strategy that aims to address leaky gut syndrome.

In her website, Dr. Ballantyne outlines the major difference between the two diets: while the AIP diet takes on a similar nutrients-first approach to food selection to other diets, it also focuses on avoiding the types of food that could indirectly trigger inflammation.

The Principles Behind the Diet

In general, paleo diet rejects many of the foods that were only commonly available after the invention of agriculture. This not only includes all processed foods but also sugar, grains, and dairy products. Some of the foods commonly eaten in the paleo diet include the following:

Lean meats

Fish

Vegetables

Seeds and nuts

Fruits

Oils derived from nuts and fruits

As a variant of the paleo diet, the AIP diet follows similar restrictions, but adds more foods and forbids others. The foods encouraged or restricted are based on how they affect the gut lining. By cutting back on food that irritates the gut lining, you allow your gut to heal naturally and bring your intestinal gut flora back into balance.

Among the foods to avoid in this diet include eggs, legumes, alcohol, artificial sugar substitutes, vegetables and fruits from the nightshade family (such as potatoes, chili peppers, eggplants, and tomatoes), coffee, and chocolate. In addition, you may need to abstain from specific medications, such as nonsteroidal anti-inflammatory drugs and supplements that incorporate chlorella, spirulina, and other blue green algae.

Some of the foods encouraged in this diet plan include the following:

Non-seed herbs (such as oregano, basil, rosemary, and mint)

Offal and organ meats

Bone broth

Sweet potatoes

Coconut milk

Green tea and non-seed herbal teas

Non-dairy fermented foods (such as kimchi and kombucha)

Bone broths

Vinegar

Nature-derived sugars such as maple syrup and honey, in sparing amounts

Probiotic-rich foods

Meal plans based on paleo diet are often quite healthy, due to the abundance of vegetables, and healthy fats. Findings also show that following the paleo diet offers many health benefits, including greater weight loss and a significant improvement in both glucose tolerance and blood pressure control.

Besides sharing many of the paleo diet's benefits, the AIP diet offers a host of other benefits for people with inflammatory diseases. Although research into its effectiveness is still in its infancy, scientists and patients alike have so far found positive results. One small preliminary study in 2017, published in the journal *Inflammatory Bowel Diseases*, revealed promising outcomes when people with Crohn's disease or ulcerative colitis applied the dietary restrictions in the AIP diet.

## Chapter 2 – Gut Matters

The AIP diet is designed to resolve leaky gut syndrome. Also known as intestinal hyperpermeability, the condition is where the tight connections of the intestinal tract's lining—which usually keep all but water and nutrients out of the blood stream—become loose.

This allows bacteria and toxins (dietary antigens) to penetrate the intestinal lining more readily. They would go on to infect the body, triggering rapid and extreme responses from your body's immune system. This would later lead to the immune system attacking the body itself, leading to chronic inflammation.

Hyperpermeability isn't the only issue at play, however. Imbalances between the natural populations of gut bacteria—known as gut dysbiosis—is tied to dietary choices and can lead to health problems.

Certain foods like legumes, starches, and nightshade vegetables often fuel the growth of potentially harmful bacteria, which crowd out their beneficial counterparts.

Dysbiosis is thought to contribute to other conditions, such as Type 2 diabetes, and may be a complicating factor in leaky gut syndrome.

Plenty of preliminary evidence supports the link between gut health and inflammation. Studies made in 2012, for instance, suggest that the type of bacteria common in the gut—which is influenced by diet—may contribute to inflammatory and autoimmune diseases. Another study in 2014 suggests that inflammation affects the functions of the gut wall, which can be worsened by food allergies that irritate the intestinal lining.

Duration

The AIP diet is among the most challenging to stick to due to how restrictive it is. Thus, it is usually not meant to be permanent.

Elimination periods where the diet is strictly followed can range between 30 to 60 days, enough time or the intestinal lining to adequately heal. However, some patients have reported sensing improvement after they have been on the diet for several months.

How long you stay on the diet is entirely up to you, but you should base this decision on how much your condition improves in the first few weeks of the diet.

One of the most important things to remember is that once you've started, you must not eat anything outside the diet for several weeks to let your intestinal lining heal. Throughout this period, you must carefully track the improvement you have throughout the elimination period. In a few weeks—or when you have finally seen significant improvements in your condition—you may reincorporate restricted foods gradually and sparingly.

# Chapter 3 – Week 1

*Step 1: Get your doctor's approval before undertaking the diet.* To ensure that your body can adapt to these new meal plans, ask your doctor for your specific nutritional needs and if there are no medical contraindications against following the AIP diet. Likewise, ask if there are any other foods that you might need to avoid.

*Step 2: Plan your meals for the week.* Good planning is the key to the success of every diet. Before starting the diet, have a list of recipes on hand to add plenty of variety to your meal plans and stock up on the appropriate ingredients. Your meal plans should incorporate not only a variety of main dishes but also occasional snack foods for when you feel like munching on something. In Chapter 7 of this book, you'll find several AIP-friendly recipes for you to try out over the following weeks.

*Step 3: Purchase quality ingredients.* Always look for the best types of ingredients, such as grass-fed, free range meats and wild-caught fish. When selecting meats, avoid cuts from factory farmed animals.

*Step 4: Organize your schedule.* You may be prepared to make the necessary concessions to make following the diet more convenient. Since finding a place that serves the right kind of food will be much too tedious, you will need to do much of your own cooking.

*Step 5: Batch cook meals in advance.* Set aside the time to cook most of the meals you would be taking to work and look for quick and easy recipes that can be prepared in bulk. For the first two weeks of the program, you would want to stick to familiar-tasting meals that are easy to batch-cook. Salads—which are easy to make and don't require cooking—will make an excellent workplace staple.

*Step 6: Keep a journal of your progress.* Your doctor may also recommend cataloging all the meals you've eaten in a journal to help you pinpoint any patterns and triggers in your meal plan. You may also report the intensity of pain that you've experienced since you began the diet. Besides instances of pain and other physical symptoms, you should also take note of your mood, energy levels, and sleeping habits throughout the diet.

*Step 7: Seek the advice of a dietician.* You can never go wrong with expert opinion. Discuss your food options with a dietician to help refine your meal plans when taking this diet and to ensure that your intake of calories and micronutrient are sufficient over the coming weeks.

*Step 8: Set an end goal.* Having a set end date for your diet can help keep you motivated by working toward a goal. Mark your calendar between one and two months further down. You can always continue based on your assessment of your health over time.

## Chapter 4 – Week 2

*Step 1: Keep your diet varied.* Feel free to try out a broader array of dishes, especially those that need a little extra time to bring out their full flavor. As tempting as meat dishes are, always complement them with vegetables and healthy sources of complex carbohydrates such as sweet potatoes. Incorporate at least one or two fresh fruits per day.

*Step 2: Never skip breakfast again.* Rather than leaving home hungry if you're in a hurry, meals as simple as fresh fruits are an excellent on-the-go alternative. Smoothies can also make a delicious and effective meal replacement and are a lot more convenient to consume on the road.

*Step 3: Improve your cooking skills.* Expand your culinary repertoire in your free time. Cooking ingredients differently can be all that it takes to add much-needed variety to your meal plans. You can watch cooking channels on YouTube for added inspiration. A recipe guide online or a mobile app can also help you find new recipes and explore creative ways to use the food you have on stock.

*Step 4: Schedule a day for culinary experiments.* Try out a new set of ingredients and prepare a different array of dishes each week. If you still find yourself pressed for time on a weekday, the weekends are the next best thing. Your downtime is a terrific opportunity to dedicate to big, delicious AIP-friendly dishes that your whole family can enjoy.

*Step 5: Waste nothing.* When cooking big meals for the weekends, be sure to save any leftovers to pack for work the following workday. These will help take some of the hassle out of preparing your meals for the next day and save you money.

*Step 6: Pay attention to possible food allergies.* Review your food journal and see if you've found any unusual patterns of discomfort tied to eating any specific food. If you found anything in your records that point to a food allergy, be sure to alert your doctor. Avoid or replace any ingredients that trigger or worsen any inflammation you may have had, and discuss anything unusual with your physician.

*Step 7: Carefully plan your fitness programs.* Regular physical activity stimulates the production of endorphins and helps manage weight—both excellent ways to manage chronic pain. Always seek the advice of your doctor before undertaking an exercise program. Plan your meals accordingly to provide you with enough energy to finish your workout.

*Step 8: Get a support group.* Like-minded individuals can encourage you to stay on track. Finding a group of AIP dieters can not only help you get invaluable knowledge with experienced individuals but also win you a few new friends who you can rely on for mutual support.

# Chapter 5 - Week 3

*Step 1: Substitute more ingredients.* Try out ingredients and recipe substitutions that you haven't thought of before. Recipes that usually call for noodles made of grains, for instance, can instead use vegetable noodles (see our recipe guide in Chapter 7 for ramen that uses zucchini noodles). This way, you can incorporate some of the recipes you used to know and adapt them to your new diet.

*Step 2: Try new foods.* Certain foods, like offal and organ meats, aren't usually very popular, but they are one of the many types of meet recommended in the AIP diet, which recommends eating up to five portions of it each week. Find an organ meat dish you might want to try. Go shopping for new and unusual vegetables and fruit see what you come to like.

*Step 3: Try unconventional flavors.* As your body gets used to the new diet and you get better at preparing salads and other quick meals, you may want a break from routine. Don't be afraid to try out unconventional food combinations. Bacon, for instance, can go with a variety of healthy fruits and vegetables such as peaches and avocado. Who knows? You might discover new favorites you'd never thought you'd love.

*Step 4: Make your own recipes.* Now is the time to experiment and get out of your comfort zone. Don't be afraid to shake things up in the kitchen and play around with your ingredients and techniques. When you find a winning recipe, be sure to list it down for future reference.

*Step 5: Make snack foods ahead of time.* Preparing your own snacks is an excellent way to satisfy your cravings while still strictly adhering to your diet goals. With a little creativity, you can transform several AIP-safe ingredients into delicious sweet and savory snacks to help tide you over between meals.

# Chapter 6 – Week 4 and beyond

*Step 1: Maintain your diet.* By now, careful planning would have helped you commit the diet plan to habit. Just keep at it. You may not see or feel the results right away, but you're still making progress toward your health. Encourage yourself by reading the progress you've made in the past few weeks. Your end goal could be the last day of the elimination period, or you could keep going afterward.

*Step 2: Adjust your diet as necessary.* If you've sought help from a dietician, be sure to ask their advice on improving and varying your meal plans. A varied diet keeps you from getting tired of routine, which is critical if you want to stick to the diet in the long run.

*Step 3: Review your progress.* Schedule an appointment with your doctor to have your health and wellness goals assessed. Your physician would be able to answer any questions you have and assess whether your dietary choices are leading to real improvements in managing your condition in the long term.

*Step 4: Add other foods, but only sparingly.* It's been almost a month since you started the diet, and if you've managed to be faithful at this point, your gut will be on the way to recovery. You may gradually add sparing amounts of restricted food in intervals of 24 to 72 hours. Take note how your body responds to the new ingredients during that time. As your diet winds down, introduce the once-restricted foods one at a time, and eat them in moderation moving forward.

# Chapter 7- Selected Recipes

## Instant Pot Bone Broth

*Ingredients*

- 1 Instant Pot
- 4 whole celeries, ribbed
- 3 whole carrots, halved
- 1 onion, sliced in half
- 3 to 4 lbs. grass-fed beef bones, roasted
- 1 bay leaf
- 2 cloves garlic, crushed with a knife
- 1 tbsp. apple cider vinegar
- 1 tsp Himalayan pink salt

*Instructions*

1. Put the beef bones in a baking sheet made of glass and season as desired with a sprinkle of salt.

2. Place the bones in an oven preheated to 420 degrees Fahrenheit and let them roast for 30 minutes. Flip them over and leave them for another 20 minutes.

3. While the bones are in the oven, take the opportunity to prepare the vegetables.

4. Once done, place the ingredients in the Instant Pot, first the bones and then the remaining vegetables and seasoning. Pour in clean water until just an inch below the Instant Pot's max fill line.

5. Seal the Instant Pot and leave it on manual high pressure for approximately 75 minutes.

6. Remove both the vegetables and bones and filter the broth using a fine mesh strainer.

7. Pour the broth back into the Instant Pot. You may use it immediately as a soup base or let it cool before storing it in the freezer for future use.

# Roasted Pork Chops

*Ingredients*

- 1 tbsp. Primal Palate super gyro seasoning
- 1 1/2 lb. pork chops (two bone-in chops, about 3/4 lb. each)
- 2 tbsp. lard or other cooking fat of choice
- Fresh thyme, sprigs
- 2 tbsp. Tin Star cultured ghee
- 1/4 tsp sea salt
- 2 cloves garlic, crushed

*Instructions*

1. Bring the pork chops to room temperature for about 15 to 20 minutes before cooking.
2. Douse the chops on all sides with Super Gyro seasoning and leave them to rest.

3. Meanwhile, preheat your oven to approximately 425 degrees Fahrenheit.

4. Heat 2 tbsp. of the cooking fat of your choice in a medium cast iron skillet over medium heat.

5. Once the oil begins to shimmer, ensure an even coating throughout the pan by tilting it slightly. Place in the pork chops.

6. Sear the chops on one side for 3 minutes and 30 seconds, then flip and sear the other side for about 3 minutes. Flip again two more times at two minute intervals on each sides to ensure an even sear throughout.

7. Bring the skillet to the oven and allow the chops to roast for 10 minutes, flipping them once every 2 minutes.

8. Take out the skillet and place the roasted chops on a plate. Drain off the excess fat.

9. Add 2 tablespoons of cultured ghee to the skillet over medium heat, then add the thyme and garlic and sauté the mixture for 1 minute.

10. Return the pork chops to the pan. Leave them to cook for one more minute,

continuing to spoon the mixture over them for one more minute.

11. Remove the pork chops from the heat and allow them to rest for a couple of minutes before serving. Sprinkle with sea salt to taste.

12. *Tip:* Primal Kitchen Avocado Oil is an excellent cooking fat for this recipe, but lard and coconut oil work as good alternatives.

# Roasted Chicken Thighs

*Ingredients*

- 12 cloves garlic (unpeeled)
- 1 tsp. avocado oil
- 1 pinch Himalayan pink salt
- 4 skin-on chicken thighs
- 1 tsp. Primal Palate super gyro seasoning

*Instructions*

1. Pour avocado oil over a medium-sized oven-safe pot. Add the garlic cloves and sauté in a medium heat for 2 to 3 minutes or until the skins begin to brown.
2. Place the chicken in a large skillet over medium high and sear them for about 2 to 3 minutes for each side. To avoid sticking, sear the skin-side first.
3. Combine the chicken with the garlic and season generously with salt and Primal Palate Super Gyro seasoning.

4. Place the chicken in an oven preheated to 350 degrees Fahrenheit and bake for one hour while covered.

## Turmeric Tea

*Ingredients*

- 1/4 tsp. turmeric powder
- 1 cup water
- 1/4 tsp. ground ginger
- 1/2 tsp. raw honey
- 1/4 tsp. ground cinnamon
- 1 tbsp. lemon juice

*Instructions*

1. Bring one cup of water to a steam in a small saucepan.
2. Mix in the honey, lemon juice, and spices and stir constantly.
3. Turn off the heat and remove the saucepan. Cover the infusion with a lid and allow it to steam for 10 minutes.
4. Let the mixture cool slightly before serving.

5. Use a spoon to redistribute the spices and prevent them from settling as its consumed.

6. *Tip:* Do not heat the water to a full boil; the hotter the water gets, the longer it would take to cool.

# Blackberry Cobbler

*Ingredients*

- 2 tbsp. organic coconut oil, with an additional amount for greasing
- 1/4 cup arrowroot flour
- 12 oz. blackberries
- 1/4 cup raw honey
- 3 tbsp. water
- 1/4 tsp. salt
- 1 1/4 tsp. lemon juice
- 3/4 tsp. baking soda
- 1/4 cup coconut flour

*Instructions*

1. Preheat oven to 300 degrees Fahrenheit.
2. Use coconut oil to grease an 8×8 baking dish.
3. Place blackberries at the bottom of pan, ensuring that they're placed evenly.
4. Place remaining ingredients in a food processor. Pulse at medium speed until

thoroughly combined and then spread over blackberries. Bake for 35 to 40 minutes or until top turns golden brown.

# Cauliflower Rice

*Ingredients*

- 1 head cauliflower
- 1 tbsp. organic coconut oil
- 1/2 cup yellow onion, chopped
- 1 tsp Primal Palate garlic & herb seasoning (or substitute 1/2 tsp Himalayan pink salt)
- 1 clove garlic, minced
- 1/2 tsp Himalayan pink salt, to taste

*Instructions*

1. Give the cauliflower a quick rinse in cool water and pat it dry.
2. Grate the cauliflower to a coarse, grainy texture approximating the size of real rice grains. You can use a cheese grater or a food processor to achieve this
3. Add coconut oil to a skillet placed over medium heat.

4. Add the onion and garlic and sauté for 3 to 4 minutes or until the onion is somewhat translucent.

5. Add the cauliflower grains and continue to sauté the mixture for another 4 of 5 minutes.

6. Flavor the cauliflower rice with salt to taste before serving.

*Tip:* If you are not strictly following the AIP diet, you may also use black pepper.

## Asian Stir-Fry

*Ingredients*

- 1/2 tsp. garlic powder
- 1 lb. chicken or beef, sliced (optional)
- 1/4 cup apple cider vinegar
- 3/4 tsp. ground ginger
- 1/8 cup honey
- 2 lbs. stir-fry vegetables, chopped

- 6 tbsp. coconut aminos
- 1 cup broth
- 1/2 tsp. sea salt

*Instructions*

1. Place all the ingredients in a stock pot over high heat and mix them together.
2. Bring the mixture to a boil and lower the heat down to medium.
3. Cover the pot and allow the mixture to simmer for 20 minutes or until the meat has cooked through and the vegetables are sufficiently tender.

## Ramen Noodle Soup

*Ingredients*

- 3 boneless chicken breasts, skinless
- 1/2 tsp. ground ginger
- 5 oz. pancetta or smoked bacon lardons
- 1 tsp. mild, unflavored coconut oil or other cooking fat of choice
- 15 chestnut (brown) mushrooms
- 3 spring (green) onions
- 2 handfuls of spinach
- A large bunch of cilantro
- 3 cups chicken stock or broth
- A pinch of sea salt
- 2 large zucchini
- 3 carrots, peeled

*Instructions*

1. Place a large stock pot or saucepan on a medium heat, then add the oil and the bacon or pancetta. Cook the meat gently until it sizzles and has turned golden brown.

2. While cooking the meat, clean the mushrooms and cut off the bottoms of their stalks.

3. Slice the mushrooms and carrots.

4. Add the mushrooms, ground ginger, and carrots to the pan and stir well.

5. Slice the chicken breasts thinly and add them to the mixture before adding the stock or broth.

6. Add in a pinch of salt and stir. Leave the mixture to gently simmer for about 5 minutes.

7. Meanwhile, use a spiralizer to make noodles out of the zucchini to the thickness of your choice.

8. Take a piece of chicken out of the pan to check if it is thoroughly cooked, then place it back to continue cooking.

9. Add in both the spinach and the noodles and stir the mixture thoroughly. Let the noodles, meat, and vegetables cook for

another 2 minutes or until the zucchini has started to tenderize.

10. Place the green onion snips into the pot and stir them in.

11. Using tongs, remove the chicken, zucchini noodles, and vegetables, and evenly distribute them between the serving bowls, then pour in a few scoops of broth with a ladle.

12. Rip up the washed cilantro into smaller bunches. Use these as a garnish for your noodle soup. Serve the soup immediately while hot.

## Green Curry Paste

*Ingredients*

- 9 cloves garlic, crushed
- 1 tsp. shrimp paste
- 2 tbsp. lime juice
- 2/3 cup chopped shallots
- 1/4 tsp wasabi powder (optional)
- 1 tsp. salt
- 1 tbsp. fish sauce
- 1/3 cup chopped cilantro stems
- 1 stalk lemon grass, chopped (white part only)
- 1 tsp. dried galangal rehydrated in 1/4 cup hot water
- 1 tsp. lime zest (dark green part only)

*Instructions*

1. Place all the ingredients together in a blender and mix for 1 to 2 minutes or until they form a completely smooth paste.
2. If the mixture does not blend well enough, add water.
3. Store any leftovers in a cool place. It will keep for up to a week in the fridge and will store for much longer in the freezer.
4. *Tip:* This recipe works even better with a kaffir lime.

## Thai Green Curry

*Ingredients*

- Green curry paste (see above)
- 2 lbs. boneless, skinless chicken thigh meat, chopped into 1-inch pieces
- 1/2 bunch radishes, sliced
- 2 tbsp. extra virgin coconut oil

- 1/2 cup chopped fresh cilantro leaves (optional)
- 1 can full-fat coconut milk or coconut cream
- 2 large carrots, sliced
- 1 lb. bok choy

*Instructions*

1. Separate the leaves of the bok choi. If the leaf pieces are large, give them a rough chop.
2. Pour coconut oil over a 10- to 12-inch sauté pan over medium-high heat.
3. Place the curry paste onto the pan and cook for 2 to 3 minutes or until it has become fragrant and its color has slightly deepened. Stir the mixture constantly.
4. Add in a third of the coconut milk and continue to cook the mixture for about 3 to 4 more minutes.
5. Then, place in both the chicken and another third of the coconut milk. While the pan is uncovered, cook the mixture and occasionally stir for 10-12 minutes or until the chicken has completely cooked.

6. Add both the radish and carrots and continue cooking the mixture for another 5 minutes.

7. Place in the bok choy and cook for 4 to 5 more minutes or until the vegetables are al dente.

8. Pour in the remaining third of the coconut milk and stir lightly to ensure it gets heated.

9. Generously top with chopped cilantro and serve.

10. *Tip:* You can pour the curry over cauliflower rice (see the recipe above) or regular rice if you have incorporated it in your present diet plan. You can also enjoy it as-is.

# Salmon Soup

*Ingredients*

- 1 3/4 cup coconut milk
- 2 tsp. dried thyme leaves
- 4 leeks, trimmed and sliced into crescents
- 6 cups seafood stock or chicken broth
- Salt (for seasoning)
- 3 cloves garlic, minced
- 1 lb. salmon, cut into in bite-sized pieces
- 2 tbsp. avocado oil

*Instructions*

1. Place the avocado oil in a large saucepan or Dutch oven at a low-medium heat, then add the garlic and leeks. Cook the vegetables until they have softened slightly.

2. Pour in the chicken or fish stock. Add in the thyme and allow the mixture to

simmer for approximately 15 minutes. Season with salt to taste.

3. Add both the coconut milk and salmon and bring the mixture up to a gentle simmer.

4. Cook until the fish is tender and opaque, then serve while hot.

5. *Tip:* If you're not strictly adhering to AIP guidelines, you can also add black pepper as a seasoning.

Seaweed Salad

*Ingredients:*

- 4 tsp. fish sauce
- 2 oz. dried seaweed (wakame, arame, dulse, agar, or any mixture)
- 2 green onions, finely chopped
- 1 tsp. fresh ginger juice
- 2 tbsp. coconut water vinegar
- 2 tsp. honey

- 2 cups finely sliced cucumber
- 1/4 cup fresh lemon juice
- 2 cups finely sliced daikon radish or Japanese turnip

## Instructions

1. Mix the honey, coconut water vinegar, lemon juice, fish sauce, and ginger juice together to create a salad dressing.

2. Immerse the seaweed in cold water for at least 5 minutes or until it is adequately soft, then rinse and drain.

3. If the seaweed pieces are too big, chop them.

4. Combine the rehydrated seaweed with turnips, radish, cucumber, and dressing. Top with green onions as a garnish.

5. *Tip:* When softening the seaweed, taste test every minute or two. If the seaweed has not softened enough, soak for an additional 2 to 5 minutes.

# Chapter 8- My Review and Analysis of the Diet

The AIP diet is one of the most difficult diet plans to follow due to the number of foods it cuts out. If you had been a big eater beforehand, this will be a very difficult proposition. Sticking to the diet in the long term could be impractical or expensive for many people. For people with autoimmune disorders, however, the price and effort is more than justified by the results it may deliver. Many people who have tried this diet have claimed that their symptoms have disappeared, and a few of them continue to follow the diet as a result.

The Challenges of a Restrictive Diet

As with other health programs, the AIP diet is far from a one-size-fits-all solution. Inasmuch as it tries to remain balanced while eliminating most of the foods linked to inflammation, there is a limit to how many foods one can exclude before following a diet becomes too impractical.

In addition, AIP and other paleo-based diets can lead to a few odd side-effects of their own. Eating a diet low in carbohydrates can lead to initial symptoms associated with low blood sugar—a loss of appetite, low energy, diarrhea, and bad breath. Fortunately, these are often a temporary thing, and you can always have the option of slowly reintroducing previously restricted foods once the elimination period has passed.

Skeptics are also wary of the diet's insistence on cutting out entire food groups, which they believe is not sustainable in the long run. Paleo diet and its derivatives cut back on many readily available source of nutrients such as calcium and dietary fiber.

Medical Issues

Due to how strict this diet is, it may not be compatible for people for a variety of medical reasons. If you happened to be on a treatment program that requires nonsteroidal painkillers, for instance, this diet may not be right for you. Likewise, because AIP and other paleo-derived diets are heavy in red meat, this might not be the best option if you have high blood cholesterol. Your dietician might be able to solve this problem by suggesting healthy sources of protein such as fish as an alternative.

Depending on the current state of your health, your physician may advise against the diet for longer than a few months due to nutritional concerns or recommend bending its rules more to accommodate for your health needs. At times, the diet may not work for some people altogether.

If it does, however, it brings many benefits along with it. The diet can help eliminate your need for powerful painkilling medicines to help manage chronic pain and even put you on the path to remission. In addition, the diet is rich in vegetables, which can also help you improve other aspects of your health in the long run.

# Conclusion

Although the AIP diet can be an excellent addition to your pain management regimen, you shouldn't expect it to banish all your aches and pains at once, nor should you think that you're eating your away out of your illness. Even the proponents of the diet acknowledge that it has its limits. Dr. Ballantyne says it best. Although food has plenty of therapeutic potential in the management of chronic illness, "that's not the same thing as calling food a cure."

The diet has the potential to reduce the frequency and intensity of pain and put you on the path toward remission. Inflammation is still a big part of many autoimmune diseases, and managing this aspect without being reliant on medications can still lead you to a healthier life.

Thank you again for getting this guide!

If you found this guide helpful, please take the time to share your thoughts and post a review. It'd be greatly appreciated!

Thank you and good luck!

mindplusfood

# THANK YOU FOR YOUR PURCHASE

VISIT MINDPLUSFOOD.COM FOR A FREE 41-PAGE HOLISTIC HEALTH CHEAT SHEET

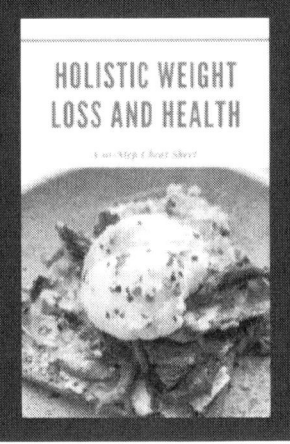

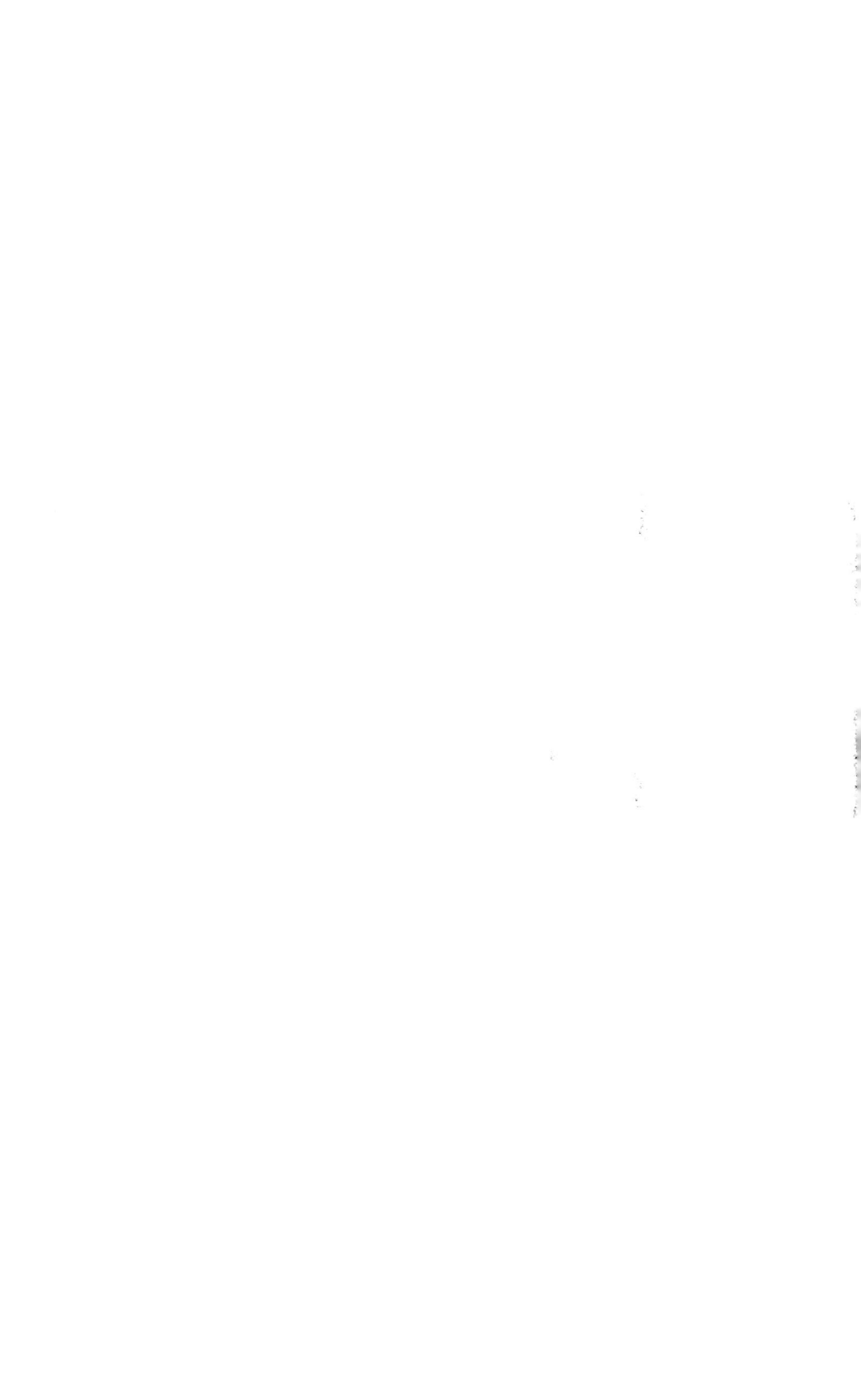

Printed in Great Britain
by Amazon